Let's Explore: Nurses Around the World Coloring Book

Welcome to "Let's Explore: Nurses Around the World" coloring book! In this book, you'll discover the amazing world of nursing through fun illustrations and creative coloring pages. Here are some instructions to help you make the most of your coloring adventure:

1. Get Ready: Before you start coloring, find a comfortable and well-lit space to work in. Gather your coloring supplies such as crayons, markers, colored pencils, or paints. Make sure to protect your work surface with newspaper or a coloring mat.

2. Choose Your Colors: Let your imagination run wild! You can use any colors you like to bring these illustrations to life. Feel free to mix and match colors to create your own unique masterpiece.

3. Stay Inside the Lines: While coloring, try your best to stay within the lines of the illustrations. Take your time and color each section carefully. If you accidentally color outside the lines, don't worry! It's all part of the creative process.

4. Add Details: Once you've filled in the main areas of the illustration, you can add extra details if you'd like. You can use different shades of the same color to add depth and dimension, or you can use contrasting colors to make certain elements stand out.

5. Have Fun: Coloring is all about having fun and expressing yourself creatively. Don't be afraid to experiment with different colors and techniques. Remember, there are no rules when it comes to coloring!

6. Share Your Artwork: Once you've finished coloring a page, don't forget to show off your masterpiece! You can hang it up on the fridge, frame it as a gift for someone special, or share it with friends and family on social media.

7. Learn and Explore: As you color each page, take a moment to learn about the different nurses and cultures featured in the illustrations. You'll discover how nurses help people in various ways all around the world.

8. Enjoy the Journey: Most importantly, enjoy the journey of coloring and exploring the world of nursing! Let your creativity soar as you celebrate the incredible work of nurses everywhere.

Thank you for joining us on this colorful adventure! Now, grab your coloring supplies and let's start exploring!

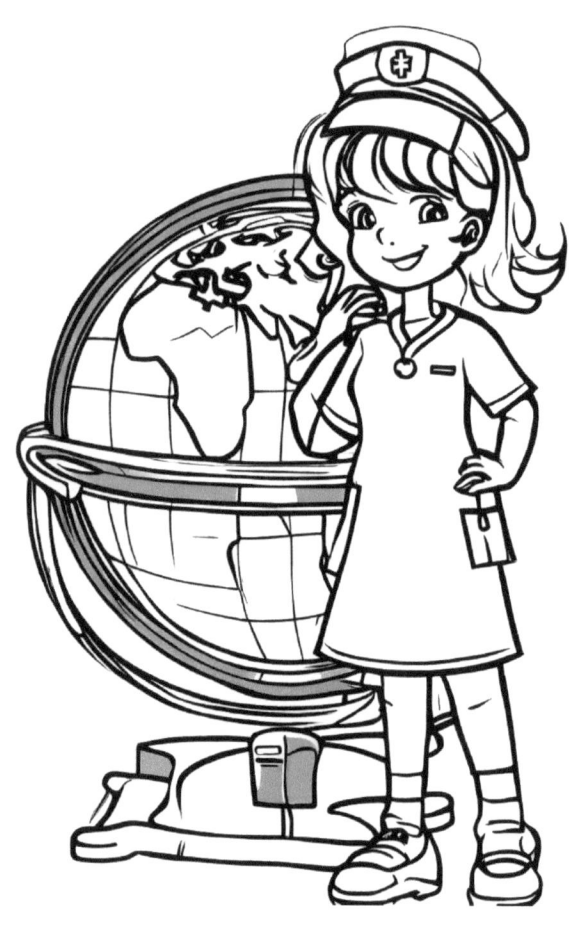

Write the name and a few words
about this nurse's story

■ ■

■ ■

Nurse around the world

"Welcome to the wonderful world of nursing! In this coloring book, we invite you on an exciting journey to explore the incredible work of nurses from all corners of the globe. From bustling cities to remote villages, nurses are everyday heroes who care for people when they're sick, help them stay healthy, and spread kindness wherever they go.
Within these pages, you'll encounter nurses of different cultures, backgrounds, and specialties, each with their own unique stories and adventures to share. Whether they're comforting a child with a bandage, delivering medicine to
those in need, or teaching families how to stay well, nurses
play a vital role in keeping our communities happy and
healthy.
So grab your crayons, markers, and imagination, and let's celebrate the amazing work of nurses around the world! Let's color our way through their compassionate care and spread a little joy with every stroke of our pens. Are you ready? Let's dive in and start coloring!"

In the bustling corridors of hospitals, the serene halls of clinics, and the quiet corners of homes, you stand as beacons of hope and healing. To all the nurses around the world, this dedication is a tribute to your unwavering dedication, boundless compassion, and tireless commitment to the well-being of others.

In the face of adversity and uncertainty, you remain steadfast, offering comfort to those in pain, reassurance to those in fear, and care to those in need. Your hands, skilled and gentle, work miracles every day, stitching together the fabric of health and humanity.

From the first light of dawn to the darkest hours of night, you are there, selflessly tending to the sick, the injured, and the vulnerable. Your presence brings solace, your expertise brings relief, and your kindness brings light to even the darkest of days.

You are more than healers; you are guardians of dignity, advocates for justice, and champions of empathy. With every act of kindness, every word of encouragement, and every touch of compassion, you inspire hope and ignite change.

In times of crisis and calm alike, you stand as pillars of strength, holding up the pillars of healthcare with grace and resilience. Your sacrifices do not go unnoticed, your efforts do not go unappreciated, and your impact reverberates far beyond the walls of any institution.

To all the nurses around the world, we extend our deepest gratitude, our heartfelt admiration, and our utmost respect. You are the heart and soul of healthcare, the unsung heroes of humanity, and the embodiment of all that is good and noble in this world.

Thank you for your unwavering dedication, your boundless compassion, and your relentless pursuit of excellence. May your light continue to shine bright, illuminating the path towards a healthier, happier world for all.

With profound gratitude and admiration,

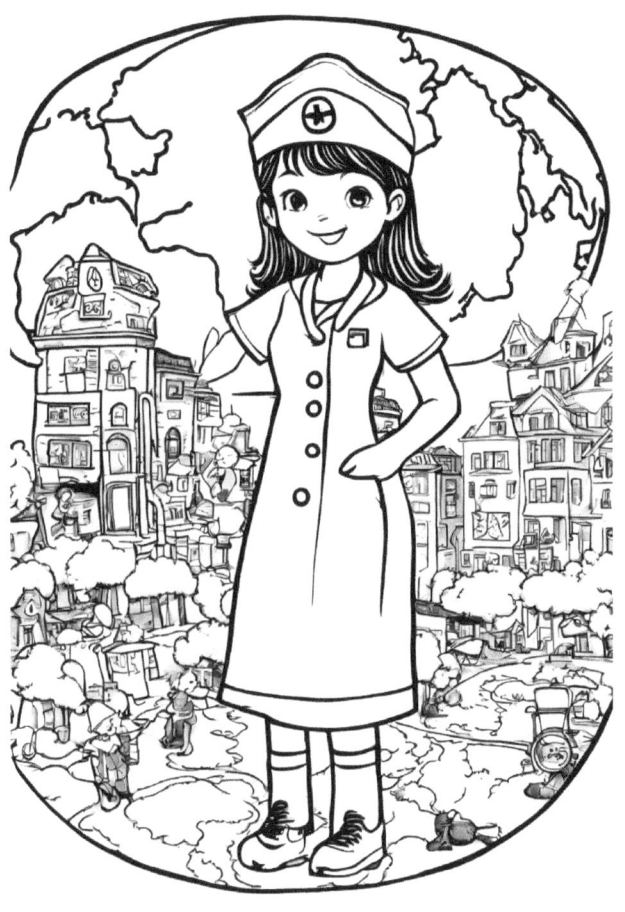

Write the name and a few words
about this nurse's story

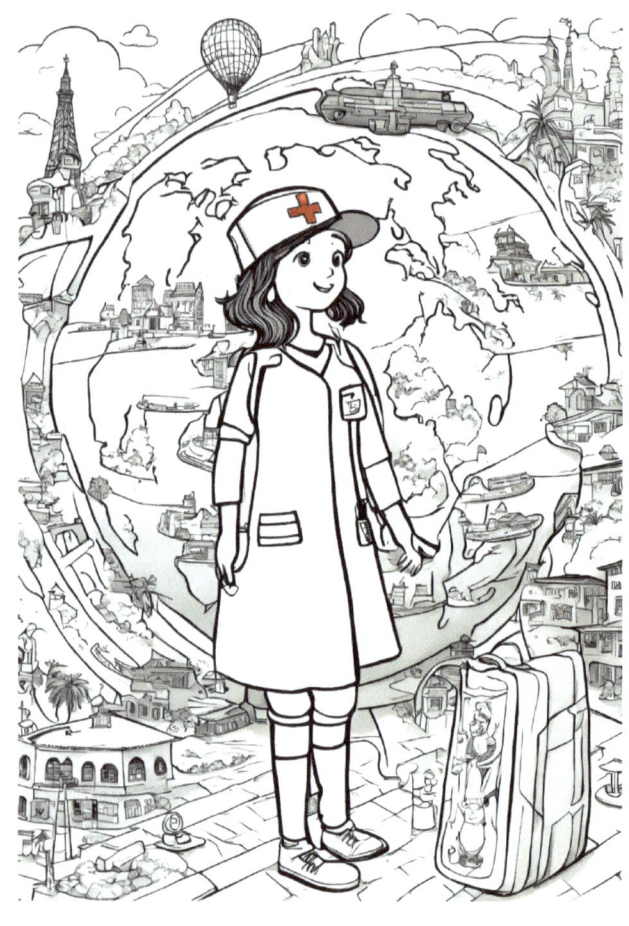

Write the name and a few words
about this nurse's story

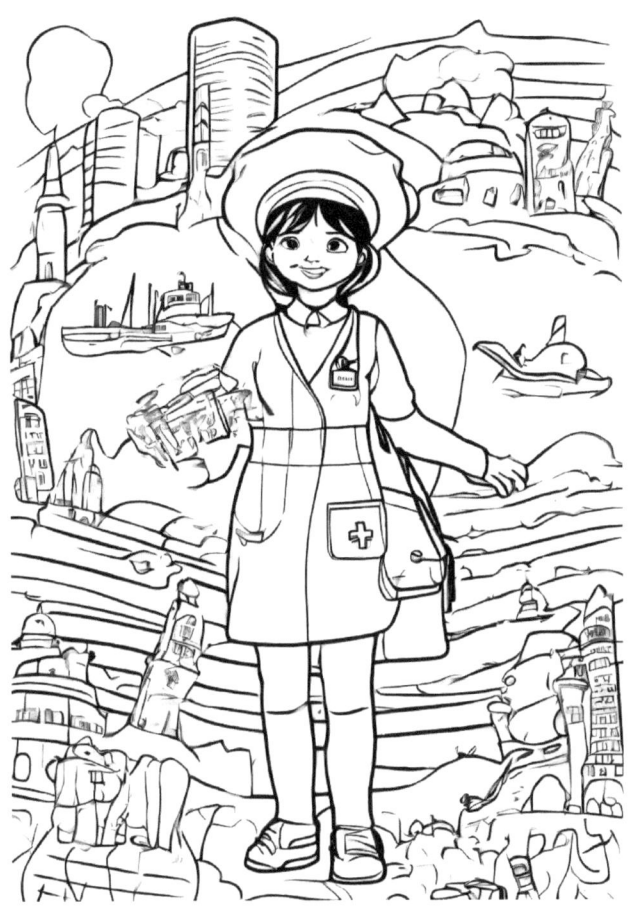

Write the name and a few words
about this nurse's story

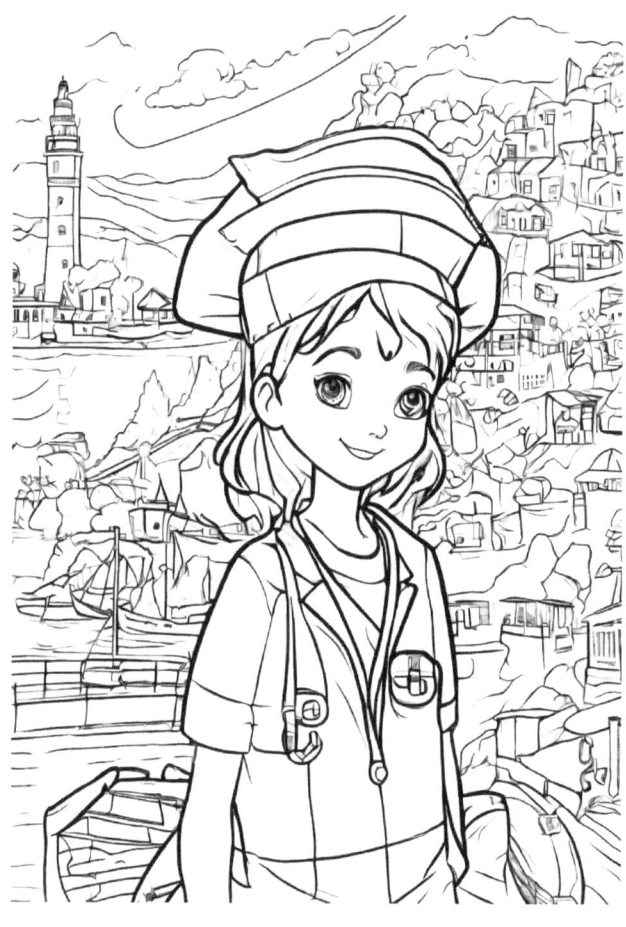

Write the name and a few words about this nurse's story

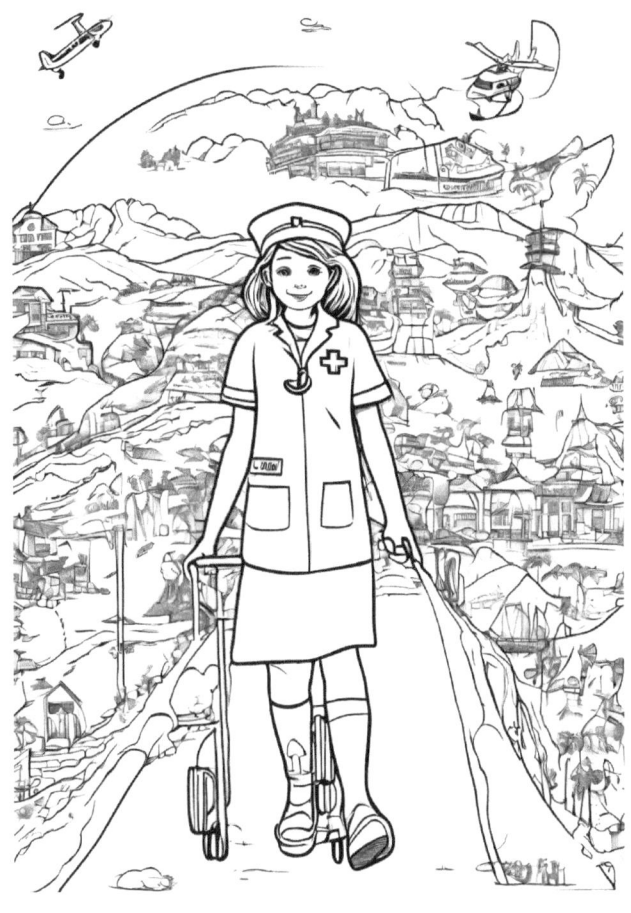

Write the name and a few words
about this nurse's story

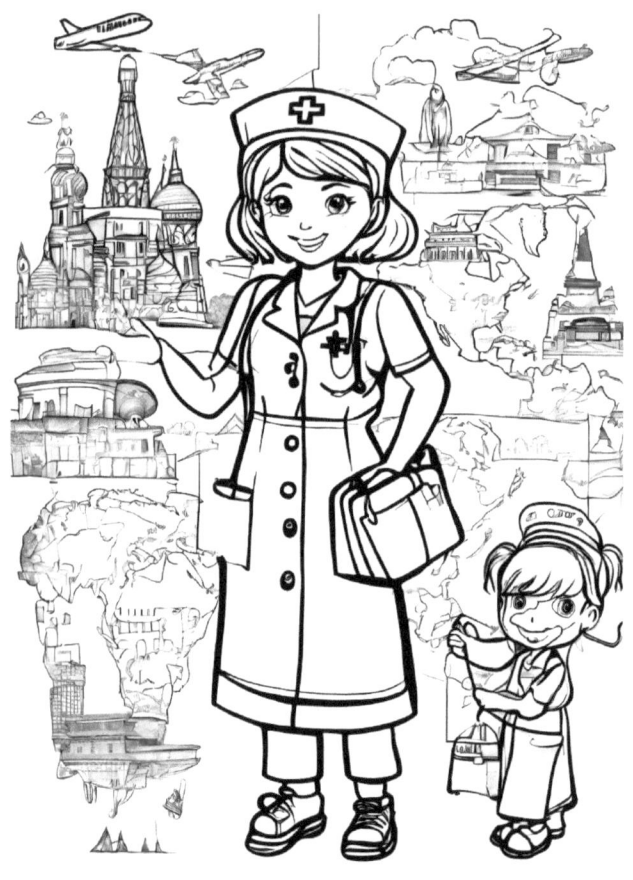

Write the name and a few words
about this nurse's story

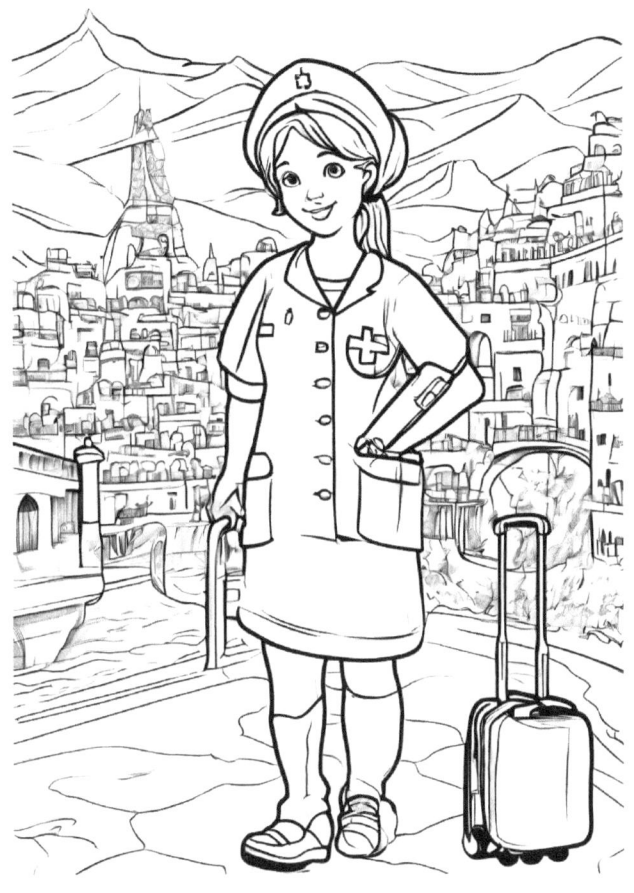

Write the name and a few words about this nurse's story

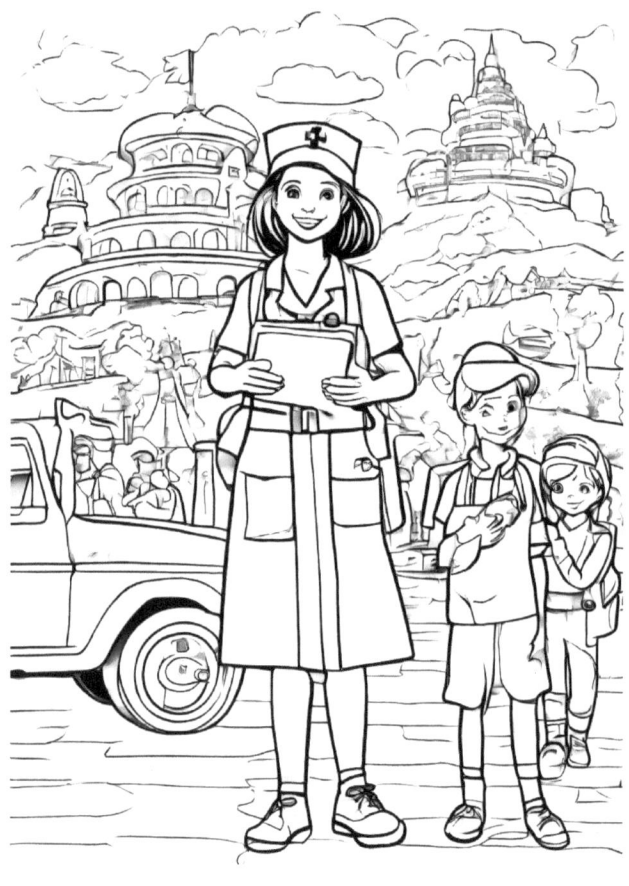

Write the name and a few words
about this nurse's story

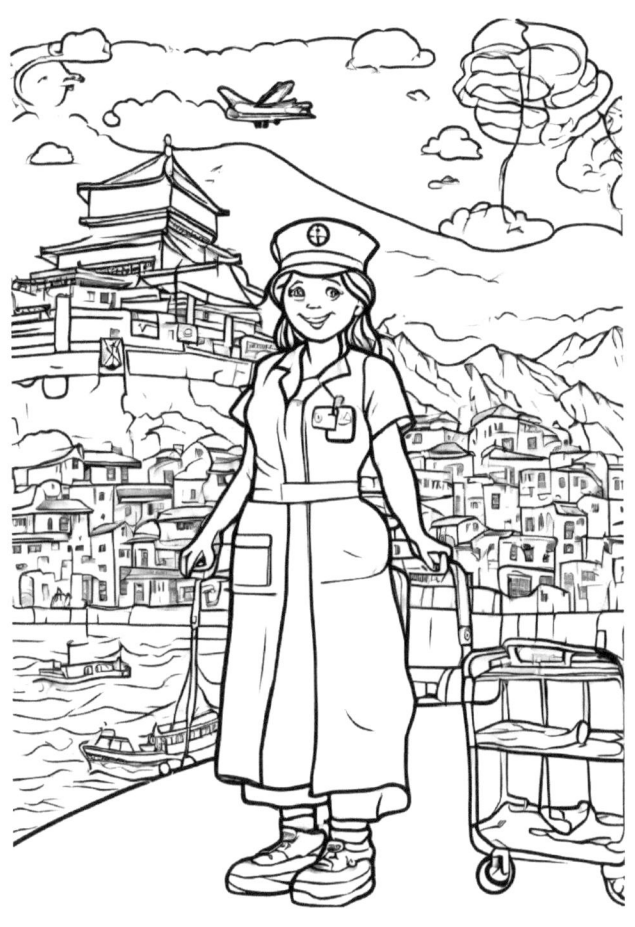

Write the name and a few words
about this nurse's story

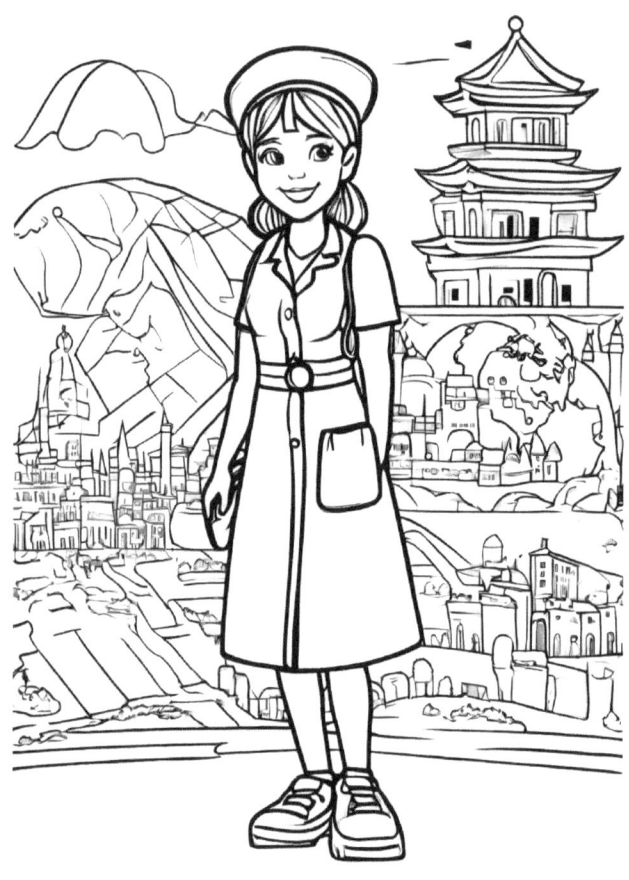

Write the name and a few words about this nurse's story

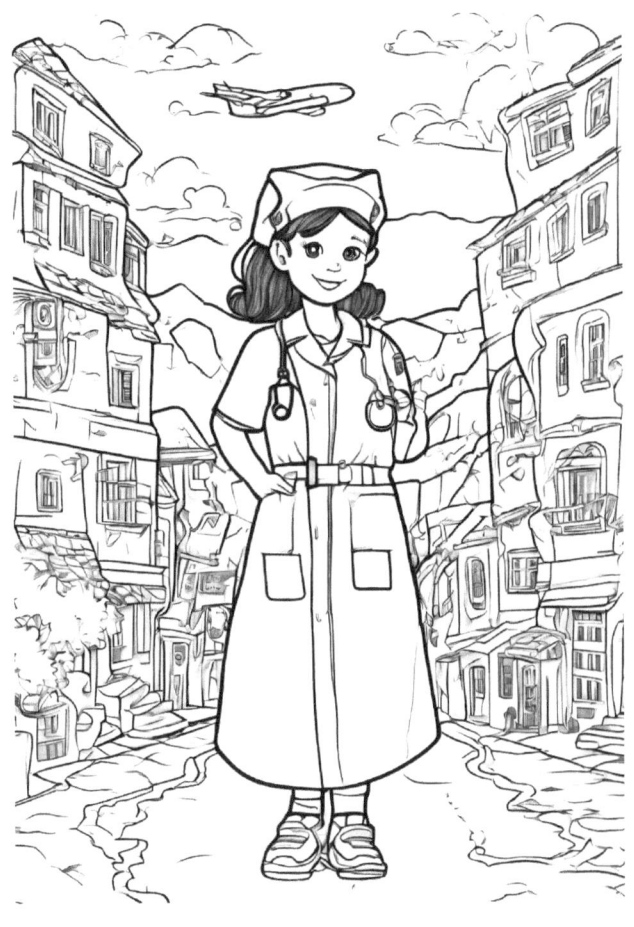

Write the name and a few words
about this nurse's story

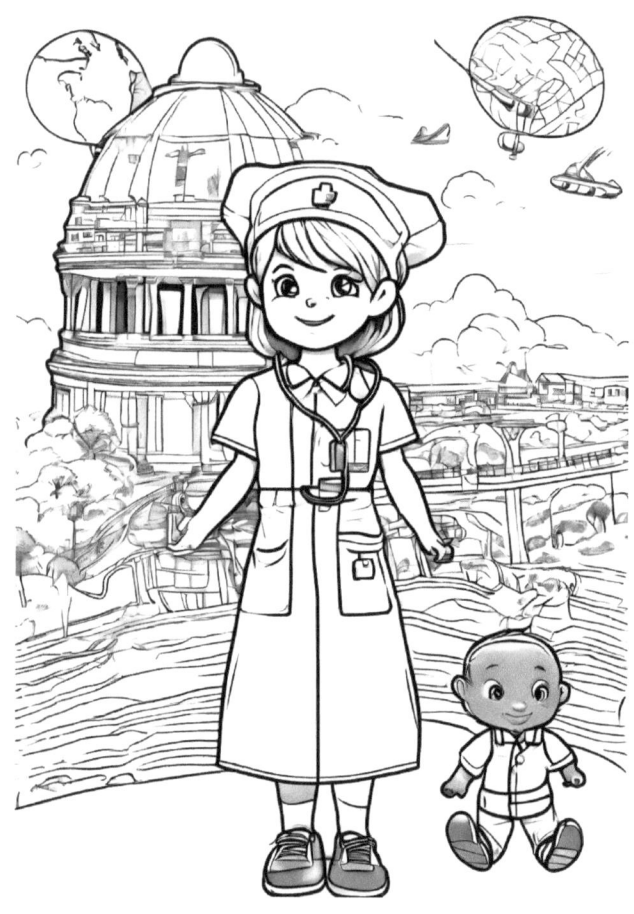

Write the name and a few words about this nurse's story

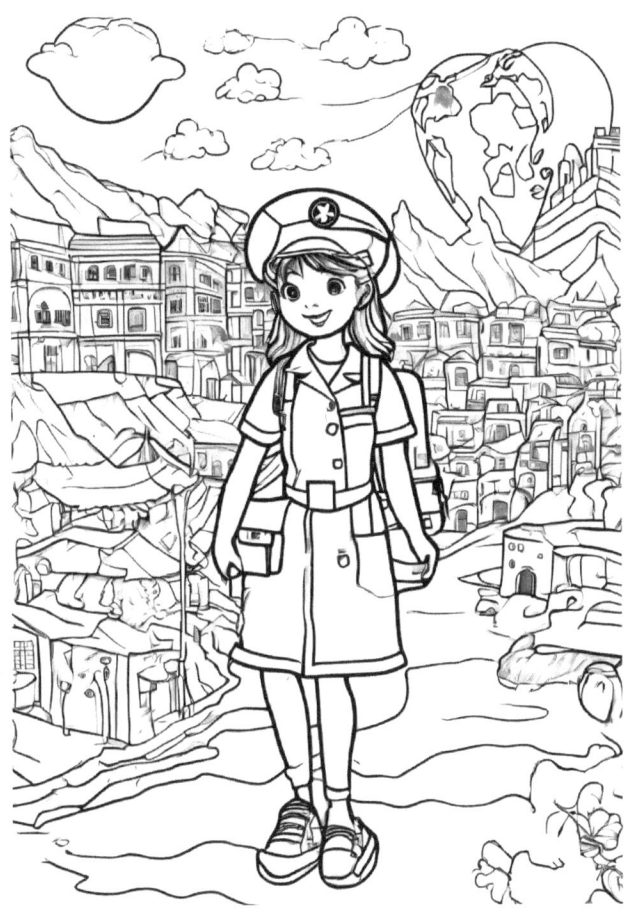

Write the name and a few words
about this nurse's story

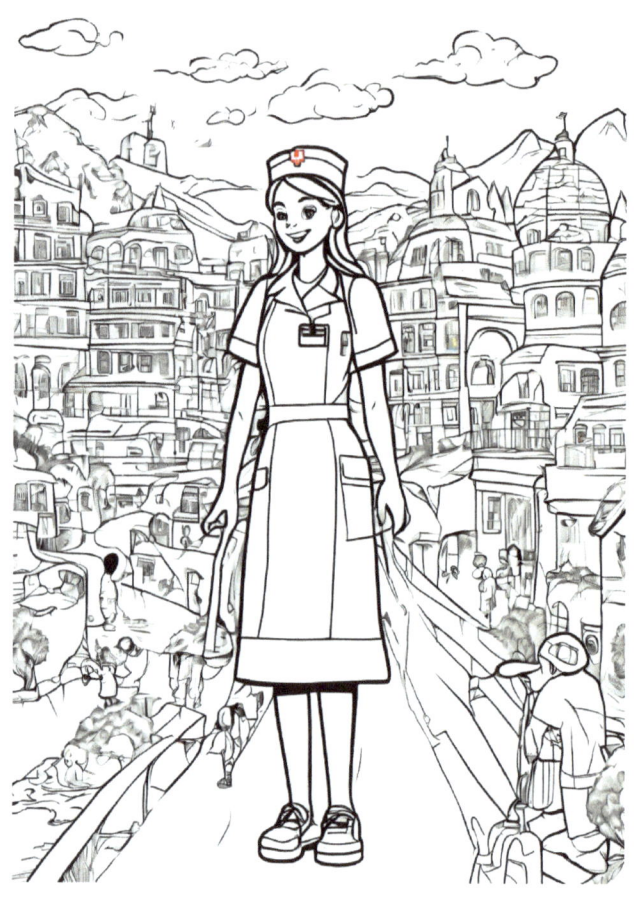

Write the name and a few words
about this nurse's story

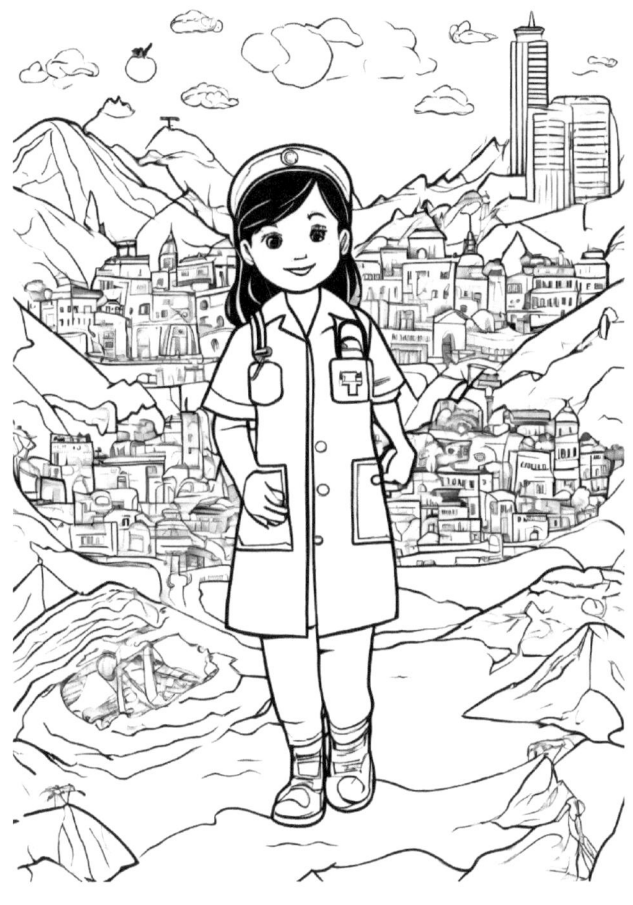

Write the name and a few words about this nurse's story

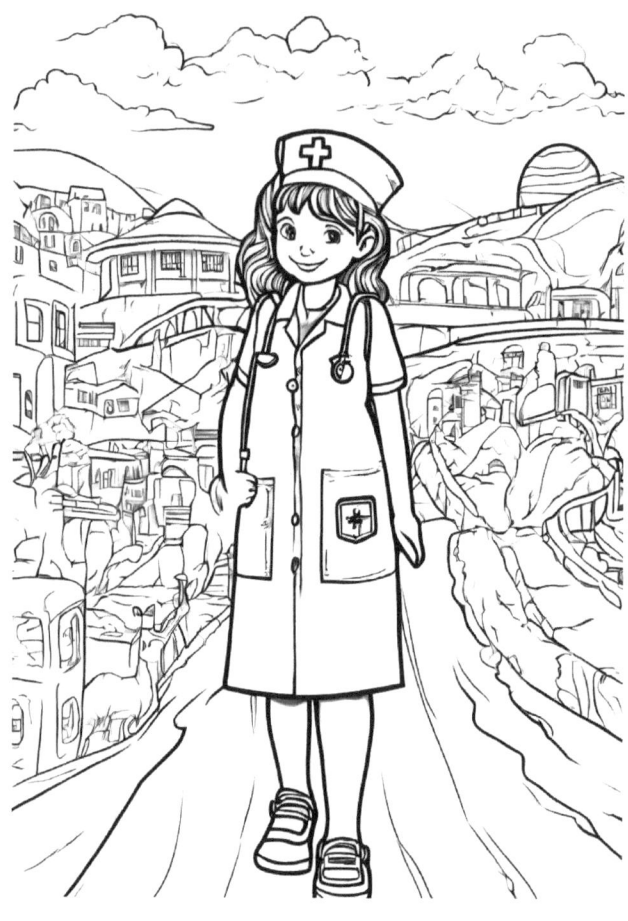

Write the name and a few words about this nurse's story

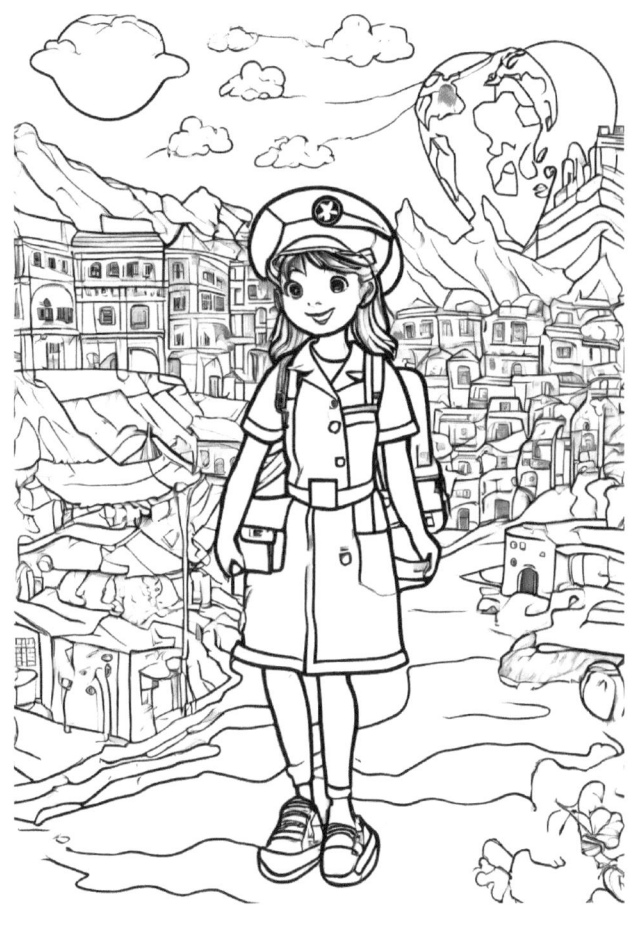

Write the name and a few words about this nurse's story

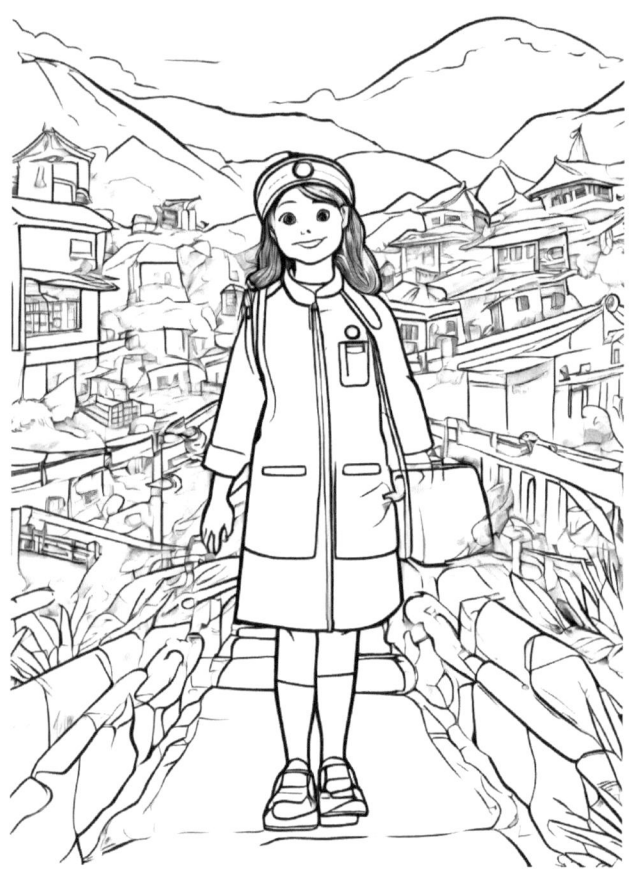

Write the name and a few words about this nurse's story

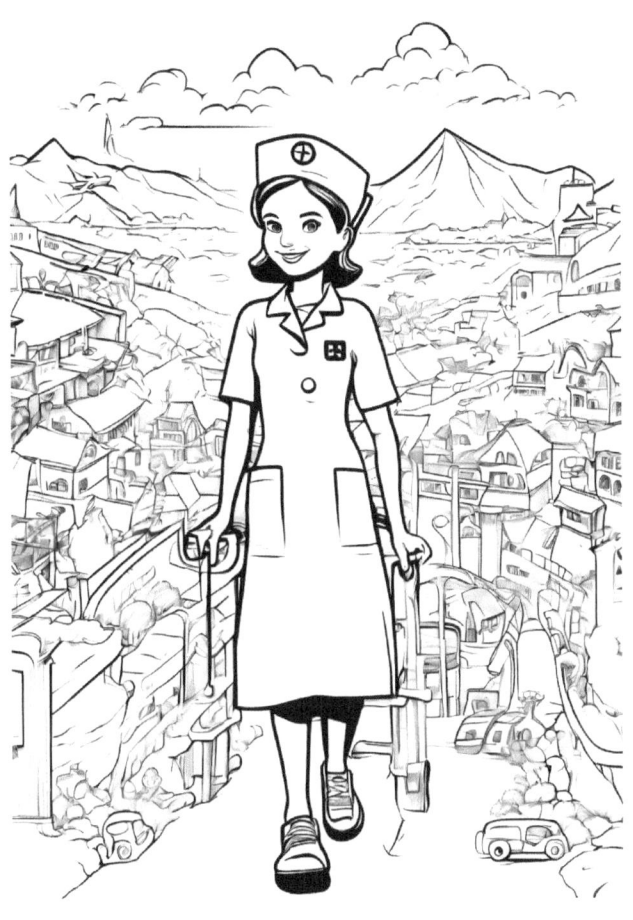

Write the name and a few words
about this nurse's story

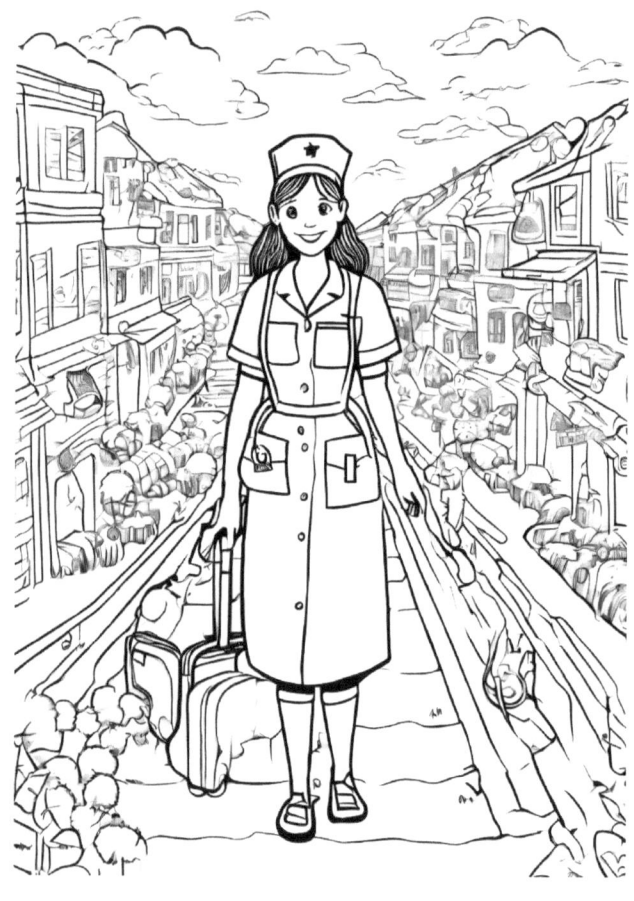

Write the name and a few words
about this nurse's story

■■

■■

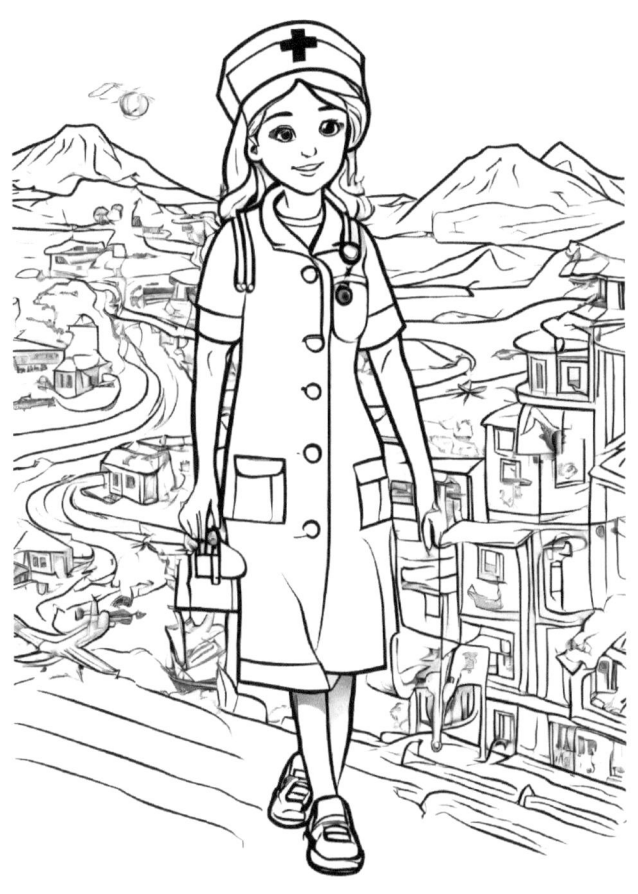

Write the name and a few words
about this nurse's story

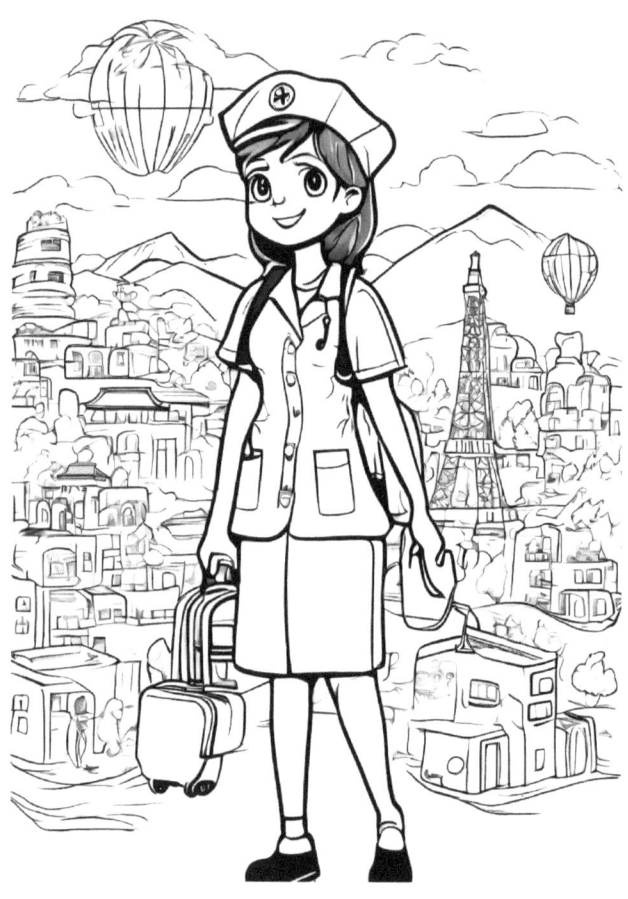

Write the name and a few words
about this nurse's story

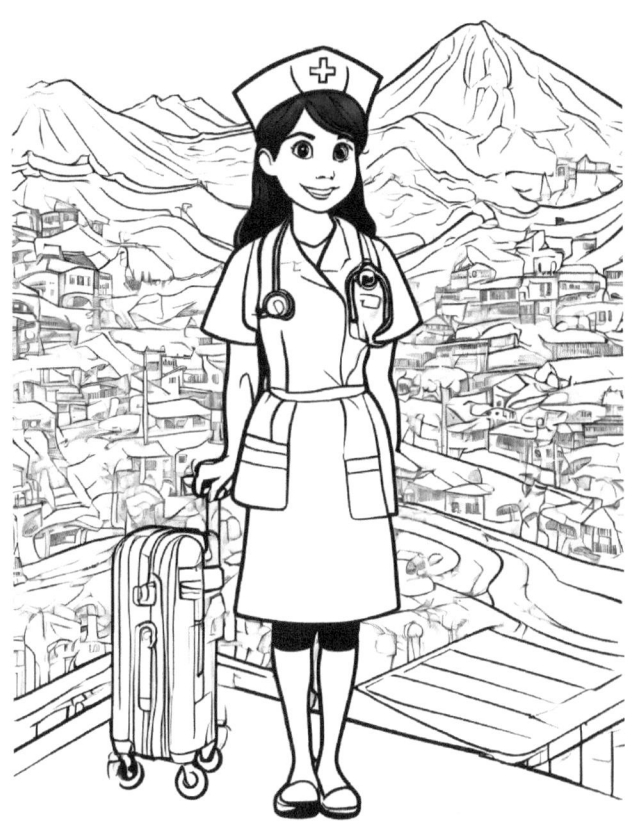

Write the name and a few words about this nurse's story

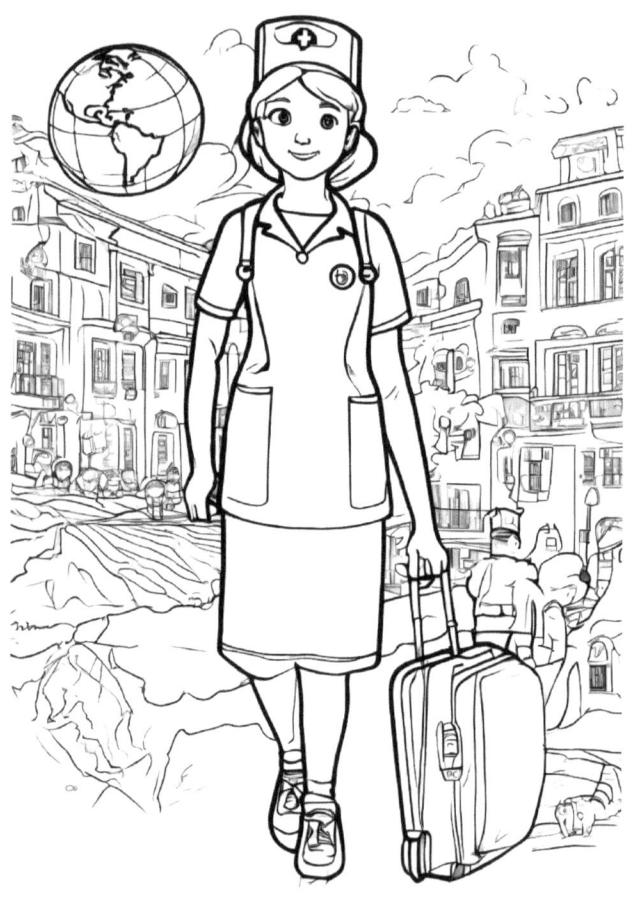

Write the name and a few words
about this nurse's story

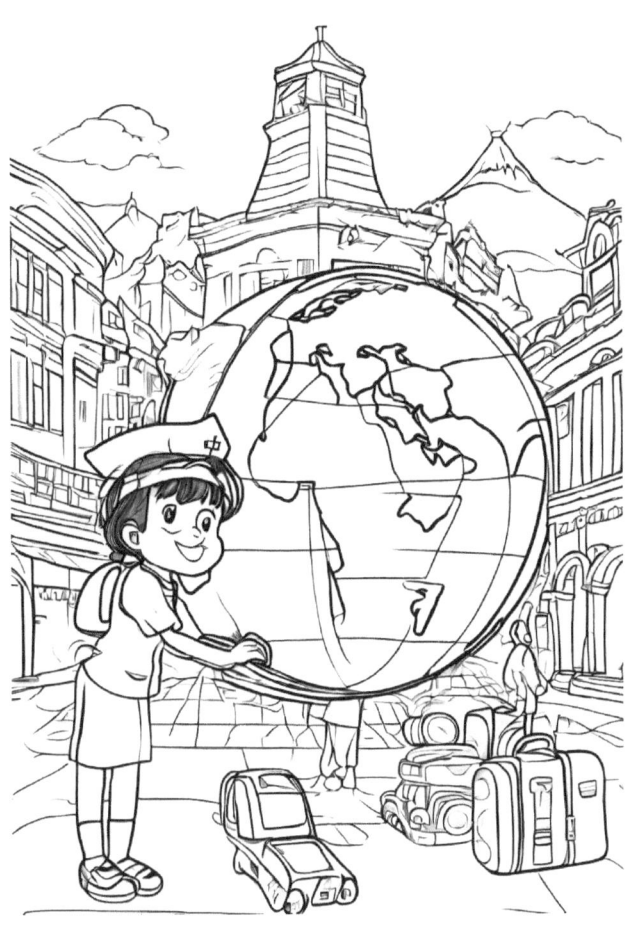

Write the name and a few words
about this nurse's story

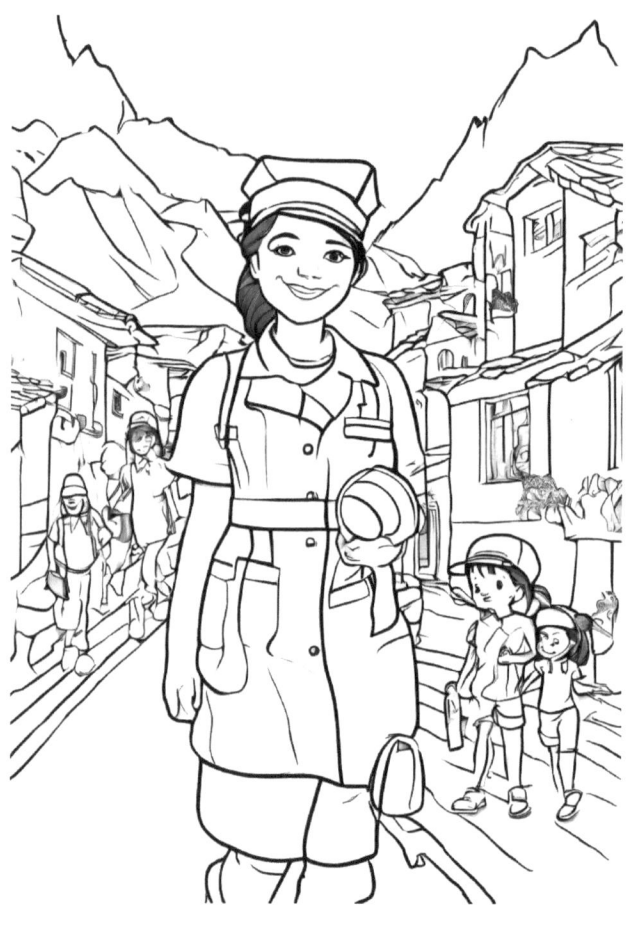

Write the name and a few words about this nurse's story

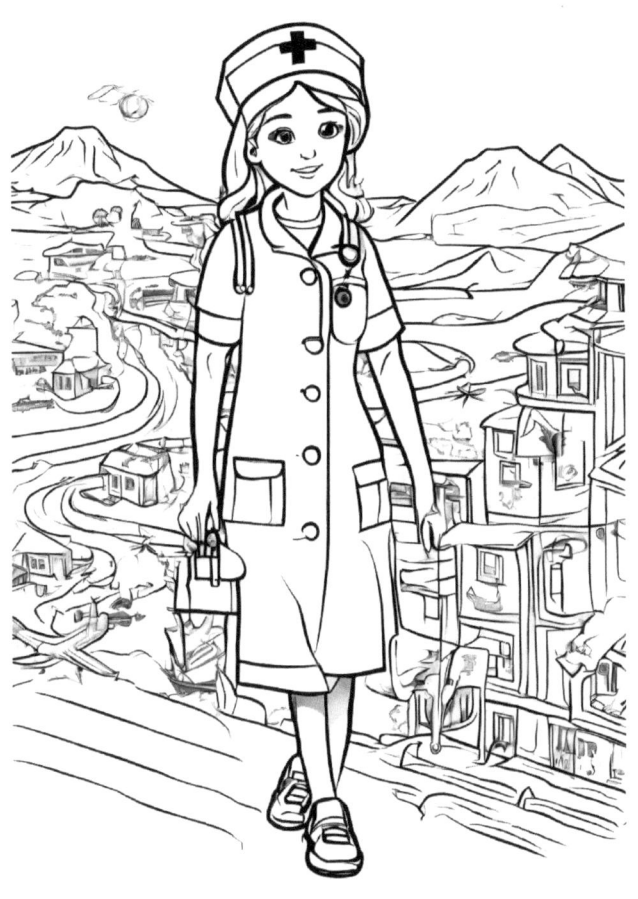

Write the name and a few words
about this nurse's story

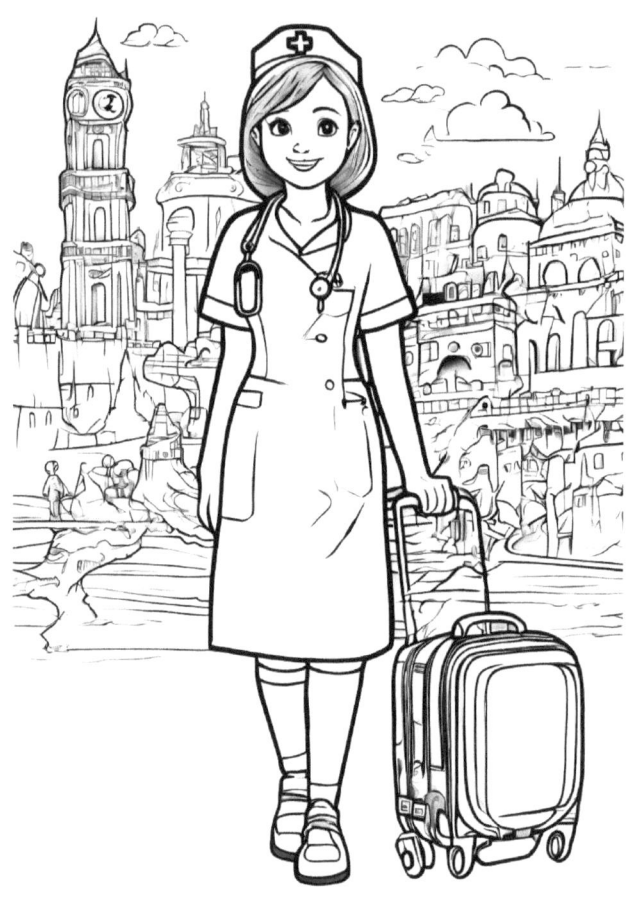

Write the name and a few words about this nurse's story

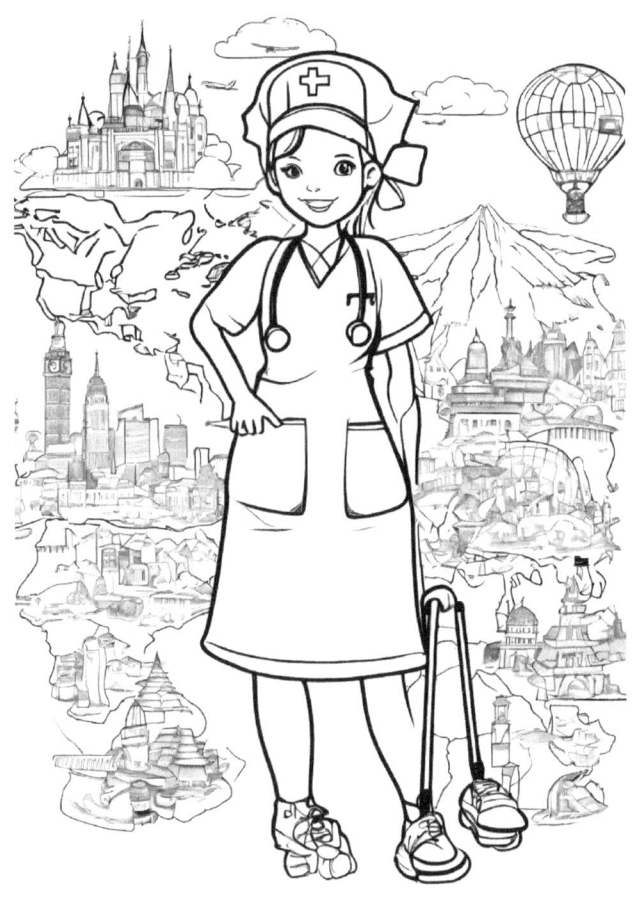

Write the name and a few words
about this nurse's story

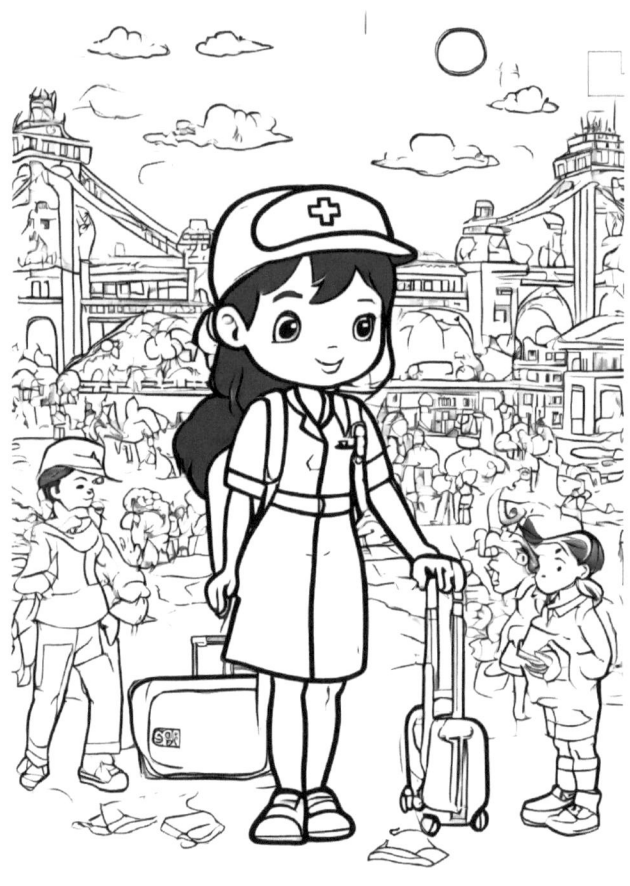

Write the name and a few words about this nurse's story

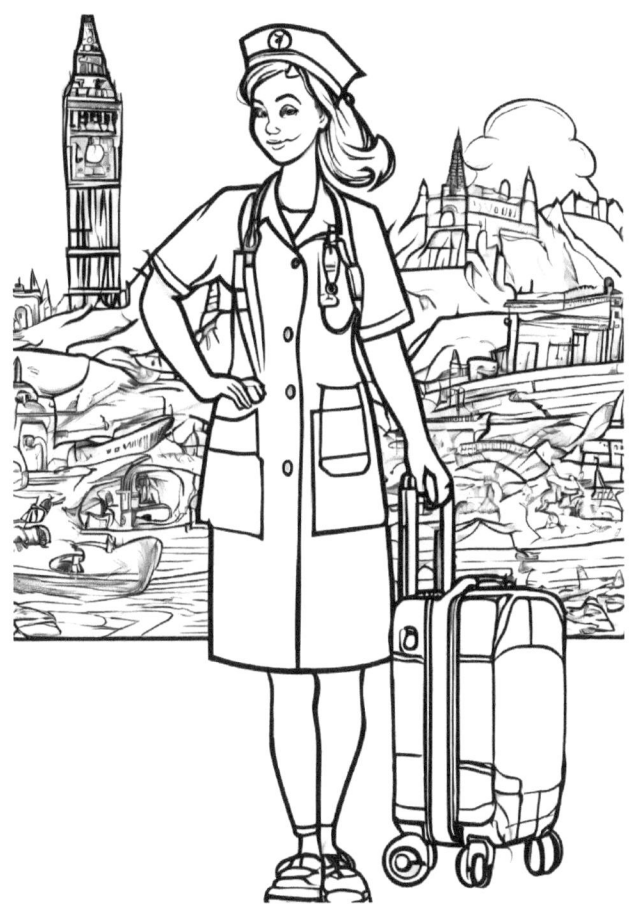

Write the name and a few words
about this nurse's story

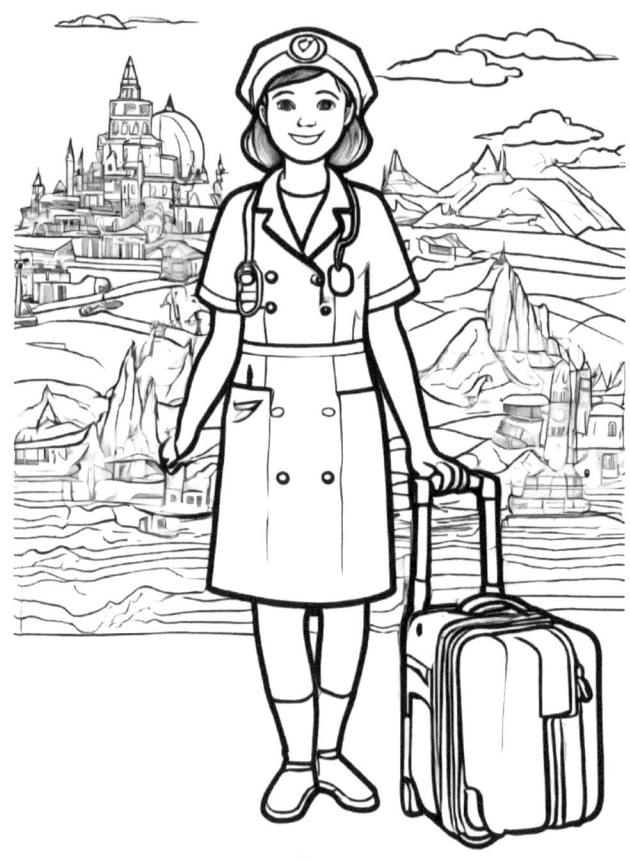

Write the name and a few words about this nurse's story

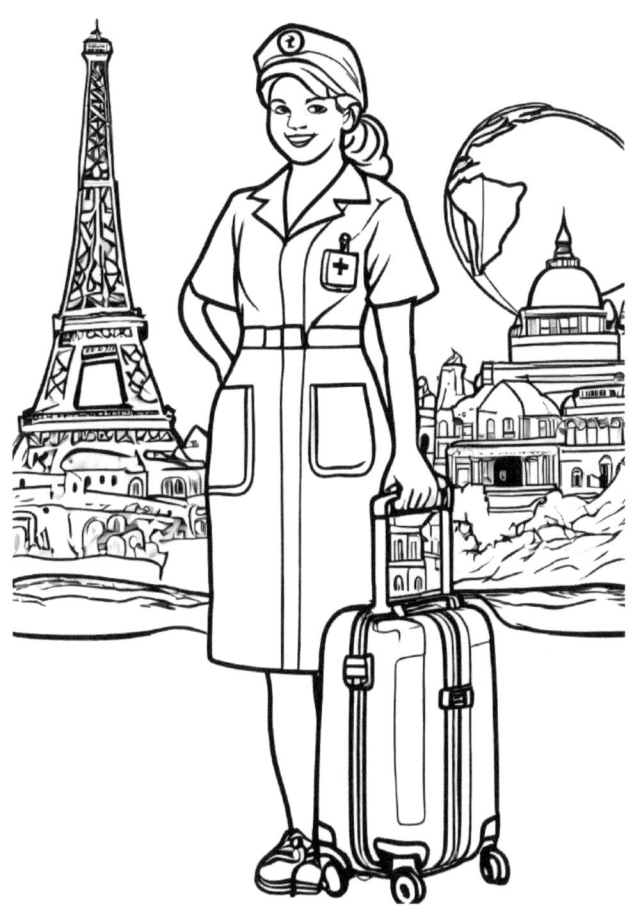

Write the name and a few words
about this nurse's story

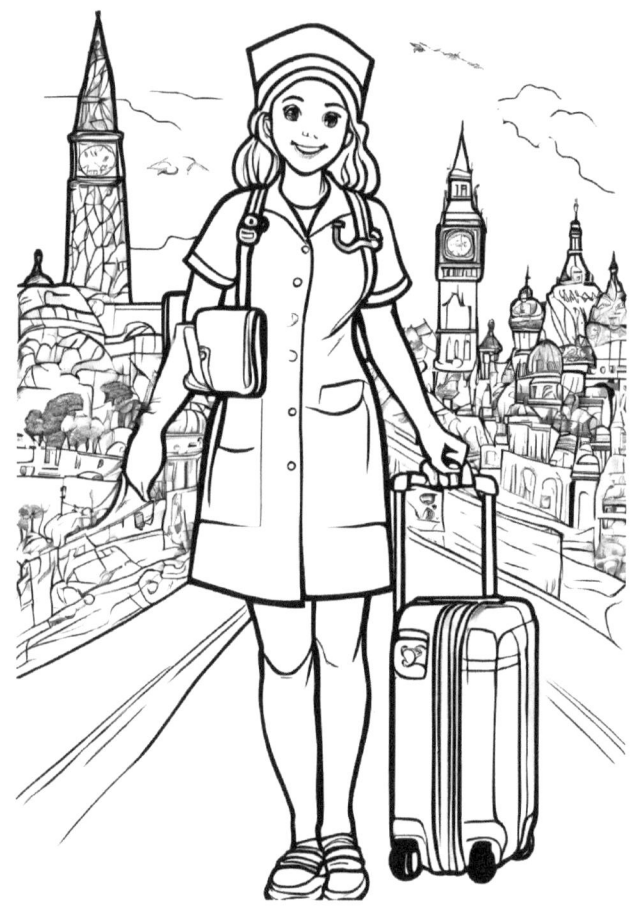

Write the name and a few words about this nurse's story

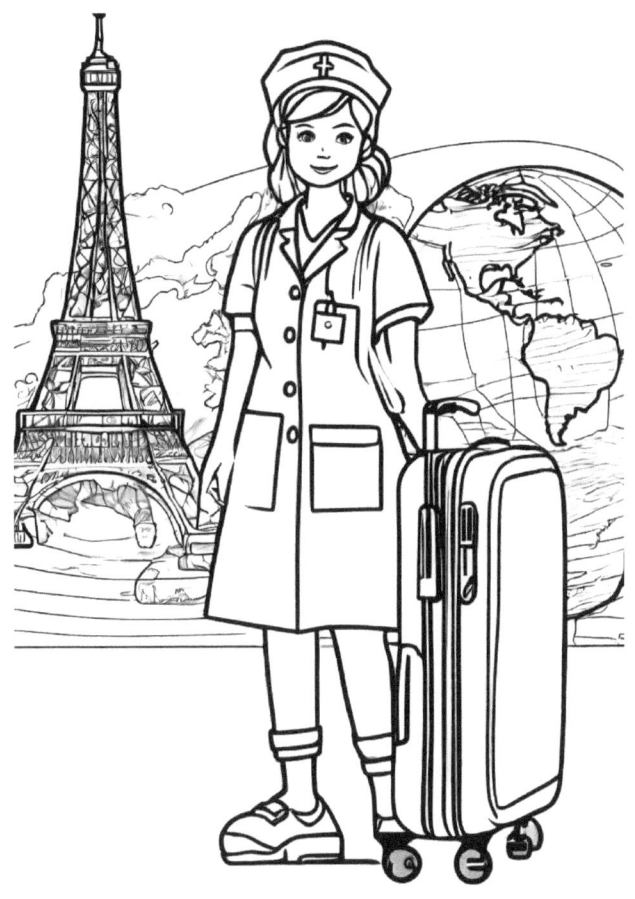

Write the name and a few words
about this nurse's story

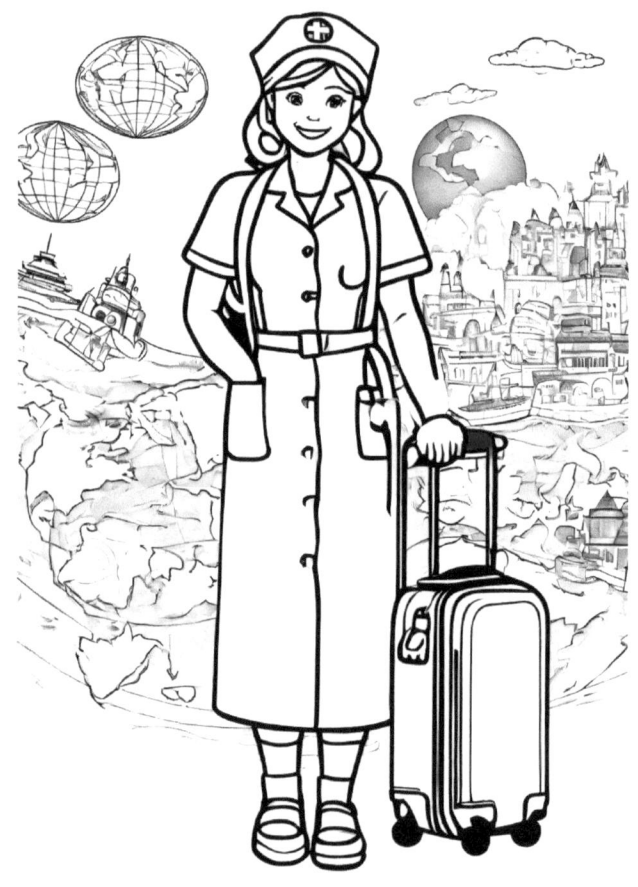

Write the name and a few words
about this nurse's story

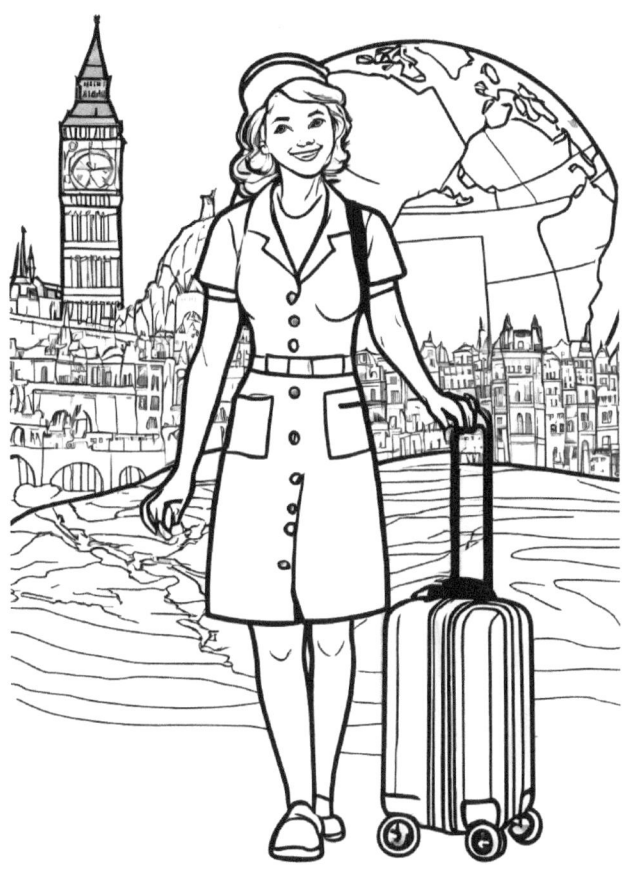

Write the name and a few words
about this nurse's story

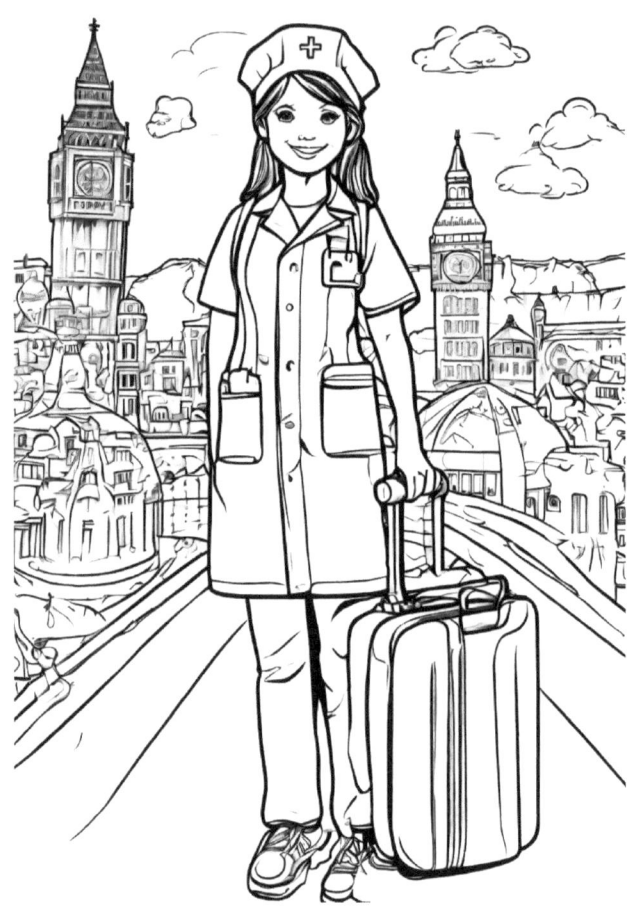

Write the name and a few words
about this nurse's story

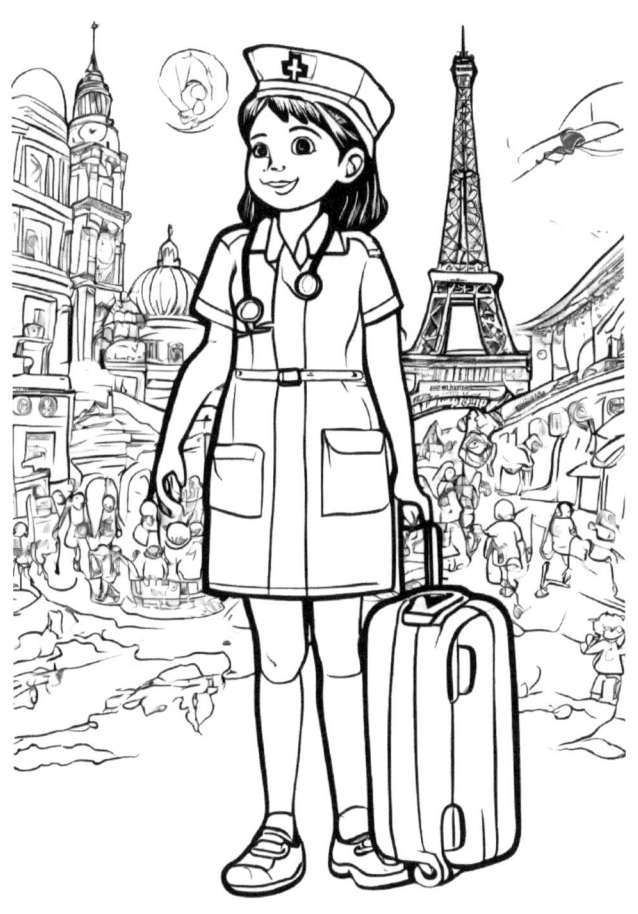

Write the name and a few words
about this nurse's story

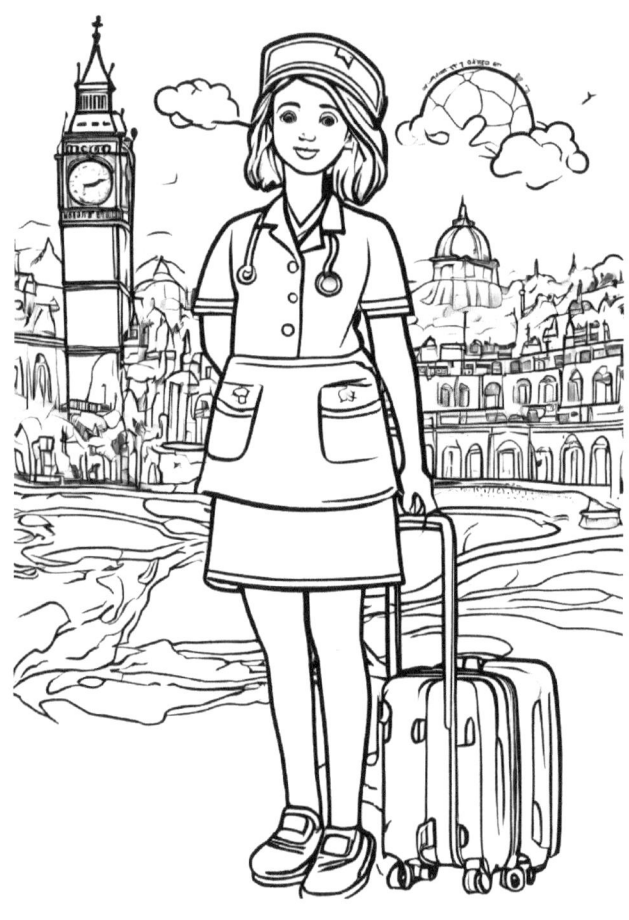

Write the name and a few words
about this nurse's story

■■■

■■■

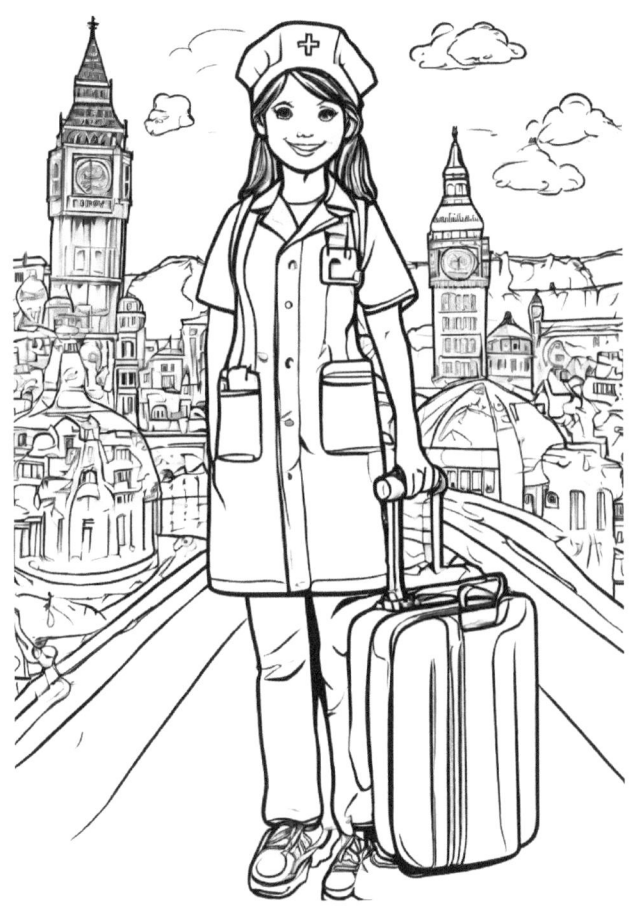

Write the name and a few words
about this nurse's story

■ ■

■ ■

"As we reach the end of our colorful journey through the world of nursing, I want to extend my heartfelt thanks to each and every one of you. This coloring book has been a labor of love inspired by my own adventures as a traveling nurse, where I witnessed the incredible dedication of healthcare professionals around the globe.
I am deeply grateful for the opportunity to share these stories with you, and I hope they've sparked your curiosity and ignited your imagination. Remember, no matter where you are or where you go, there are always heroes among us, spreading kindness and caring for those in need.
To all the nurses, past, present, and future, thank you for your unwavering commitment to healing and compassion. And to all the budding artists who have brought these pages to life with your colorful creativity, you have truly made this journey unforgettable.
May your days be filled with love, laughter, and endless possibilities. And as you continue to explore the world around you, may you always carry with you the spirit of kindness and the belief that small acts of compassion can make a big difference.
With heartfelt gratitude,

Arianna B. - Nurse"

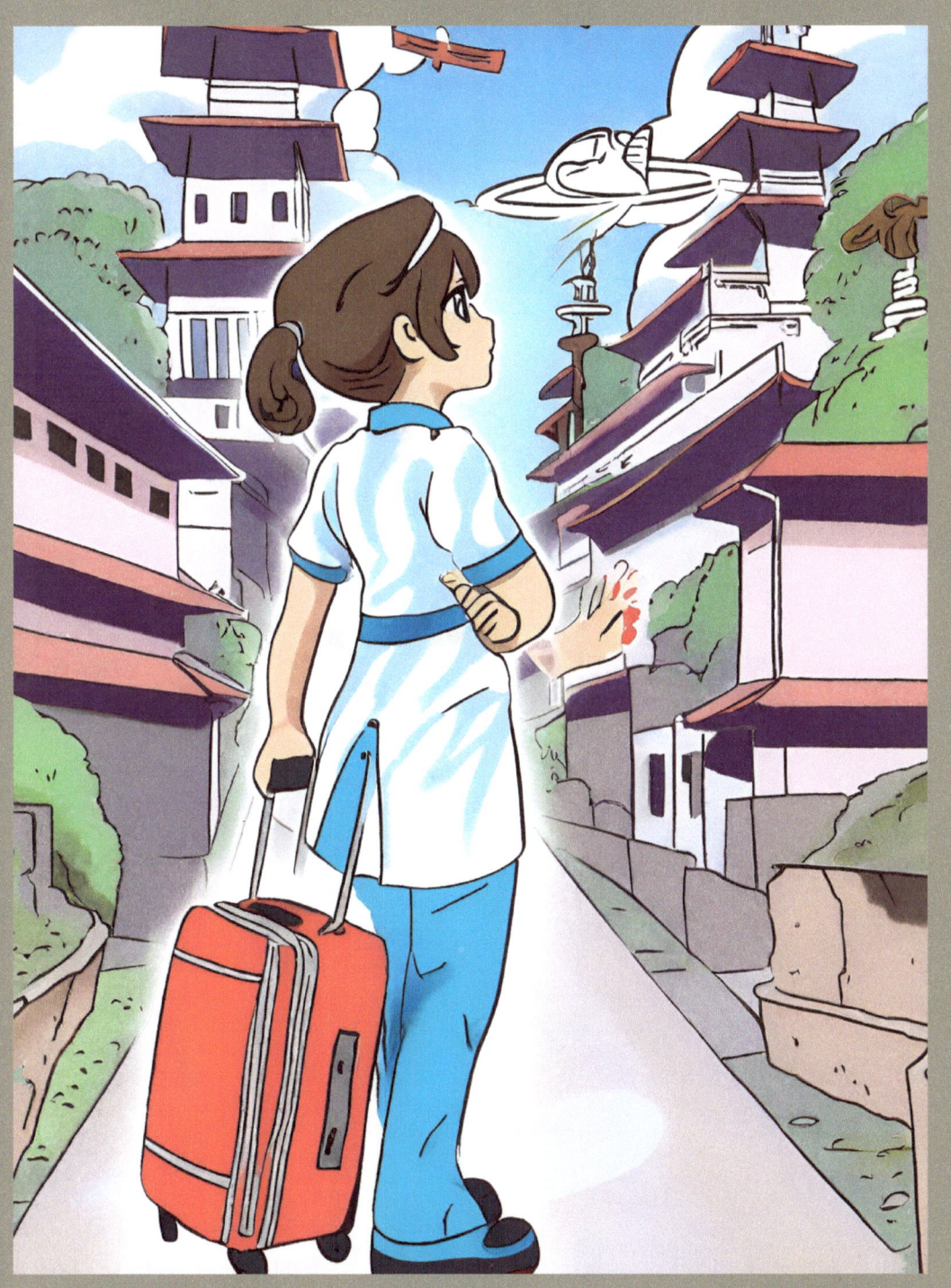

www.ingramcontent.com/pod-product-compliance
Lightning Source LLC
Chambersburg PA
CBHW040331220526
45473CB00009B/2650